Qualified in 1991 at the University of Fort Hare (B Cur) in South Africa majoring in general nursing science, psychiatry, community health nursing and midwifery, nursing people with mental health issues has been his life. Mr Vuyisile Louis Poti worked in mental health, community hospitals, mental health clinics (initial and follow-up stages) and nursing homes. He worked in various hospitals across England as a mental health nurse, registered nurse and a carer. It is that exposure to his clients that gave him the understanding of the people he was looking after and the efforts of other professionals supporting the services viz, doctors, psychiatrists, psychologists, community psychiatric nurses and dementia supporting groups etc.

This book is dedicated to my mum, Thembeka Eleanor Poti, as a thank you for her love and efforts in making me what I am today. Thanks again, Tabi.

Vuyisile Louis Poti

THE QUOTABLE QUOTES: DEMENTIA REFINED

AUSTIN MACAULEY PUBLISHERS™
LONDON • CAMBRIDGE • NEW YORK • SHARJAH

Copyright © Vuyisile Louis Poti (2021)

The right of Vuyisile Louis Poti to be identified as author of this work has been asserted by the author in accordance with section 77 and 78 of the Copyright, Designs and Patents Act 1988.

All rights reserved. No part of this publication may be reproduced, stored in a retrieval system, or transmitted in any form or by any means, electronic, mechanical, photocopying, recording, or otherwise, without the prior permission of the publishers.

Any person who commits any unauthorized act in relation to this publication may be liable to criminal prosecution and civil claims for damages.

A CIP catalogue record for this title is available from the British Library.

ISBN 9781528929592 (Paperback)
ISBN 9781528965927 (ePub e-book)

www.austinmacauley.com

First Published (2021)
Austin Macauley Publishers Ltd
25 Canada Square
Canary Wharf
London
E14 5LQ

Also I would like to thank my wife, Nolita, sons—Gcobani, Siyabulela, Luvo and Sisipho—for being patient and let me pursue this career and lastly to my new acquired polish family, Adam Sierpinski and Janina, Pysio and his wife Renata Bochnak and their sons Damian and Przemo.

Table of Content

Introduction	**12**
Chapter One	**20**
"I am Scared"	*20*
Chapter Two	**29**
"Where Is You Born?"	*29*
Chapter Three	**33**
Chapter Four	**36**
Chapter Five	**41**
Chapter Six	**46**
Chapter Seven	**52**
Chapter Eight	**57**
Chapter Nine	**63**
Chapter Ten	**71**
Chapter Eleven	**76**
Chapter Twelve	**80**
Chapter Thirteen	**86**

Chapter Fourteen	91
Chapter Fifteen	94
Conclusion	100
References	104

About this Book

The characters in this book are fictional but the events are true and quotations are taken from people suffering from dementia, carers and professionals looking after people with dementia across England. The names of the characters were given randomly and neither have significance to the people suffering from dementia nor their families.

This book highlights some of the growing concerns in Nursing and Care homes looking after people with dementia across the UK.

Quotable quotes are trying to seek and explore some of the myths about dementia and put to light that these people we are dealing with, do feel and sometimes understand. Its main objective is to enlighten the care-givers that it is not gloom and doomed, we can break through this barrier and people suffering from dementia can get the quality care they deserve and live their lives to the fullest. It aims to teach personnel to decode the verbal cues put to us across by the people suffering with dementia and respect their wishes.

They are human and they deserve to be treated as such. Dementia is a progressive disease with devastating effects both physically, spiritually and emotionally. The suffering is unbearable to be polite.

Introduction

Based on the true events these quotable quotes were taken from clients who were in care or shall I say, these are tales from the vault. This definitely poses a question to us carers, nurses, health care practitioners, families, friends and significant others. Do we take the individuals we are looking after and our loved ones for granted? Are we doing enough?

A lovely journey turned sour. Listening to promises like We will be here tomorrow mum. Listening to lies like We are just popping out to buy something and we'll be back soon. Listening to honesty that We are going to leave you mum, we are both working and the children are at school and there is no one to look after you, you are in good capable hands. Straight talk breaks no friendship. It is a bitter pill to swallow, but honesty goes a long way and lies have shorter legs. These neither make things easier for the clients nor for the professionals who are looking after them because they will always echo throughout their lives and delay their time to settle.

The promised land – flowers and smiles, pens down and gloves off, a spectacular welcome to the delight of the family and significant others. Both parties are happy with the exception of the client who is emotionally drained by the process and disorientation in every aspect. He/she is the main focus, just as the doctor has ordered, perfect, what a superb treat?

Life is a struggle, but dementia is more than a struggle. When your life is turned upside down, maintaining the balance is a big challenge. The myths surrounding the disease are daunting and when faced with this problem you really need caring, supportive and understanding professionals, care-givers, families and friends.

Dementia is clouded with loads of malpractices and mis-judgments. Tom Kitwood (2005), reflecting on malignant social psychology states that if we come close to the details of how life is lived, hour by hour and minute by minute, we can see many processes that work towards the undermining of people who have dementia.

Quoting and adding to his original work, he further stresses that the term malignant does not, however imply evil intent on the part of the caregivers, most of their work is done with kindness and good intent, and the malignancy is a part of our cultural inheritance. His list contains, with seven further added elements the following:

1. Treachery: Using forms of deception in order to distract or manipulate a person, or force them into compliance.
2. Disempowerment: Not allowing a person to use the abilities that they do have; failing to help them to complete actions that they have initiated.
3. Infantilization: Treating a person very patronizingly (or "matronizingly") as an insensitive parent might treat a very young child.

4. Intimidation: Inducing fear in a person, through the use of threats or physical power.
5. Labelling: Using a category such as dementia, or "organic mental disorder", as the main basis for interacting with a person and for explaining their behaviour.
6. Stigmatization: Treating a person as if they were a diseased object, an alien or an outcast.
7. Outpacing: Providing information, presenting choices, etc. at a rate too fast for a person to understand; putting them under pressure to do things more rapidly than they can bear.
8. Invalidation: Failing to acknowledge the subjective reality of a person's experience, and especially what they are feeling.
9. Banishment: Sending a person away, or excluding them -physical or psychological.
10. Objectification: Treating a person as if they were a lump of dead matter; to be pushed, lifted, filled, pumped or drained, without proper reference to the fact that they are sentient beings.
11. Ignoring: Carrying on (in conversation or action) in the presence of a person as if they were not there.
12. Imposition: Forcing a person to do something, overriding desire or denying the possibility of choice on their part.
13. Withholding: Refusing to give asked-for attention, or to meet an evident need.
14. Accusation: Blaming a person for actions or failures of action that arise from their lack of ability, or their misunderstanding of the situation.

15. Disruption: Intruding suddenly or disturbingly upon a person's action or reflection; crudely breaking their frame of reference.
16. Mockery: Making fun of a person's strange actions or remarks; teasing, humiliating, making jokes at their expense.
17. Disparagement: Telling a person that they are incompetent, useless, worthless, etc., giving them messages that are damaging to their self-esteem.

These are undeniable facts and are proved to have a very negative impact in the care of the vulnerable dementia sufferers we are looking after. The importance of tracking and investigating the reason for the behaviour is totally missed. We do not view the world in their context. Just have a look at this: Sweet-Potato is nursed in bed. She has not been feeling well for the past two days. She has lost weight and has lost appetite. When her daughter Pauline is in, she eats and drink well. She does not feel comfortable, though but she does force a smile. The difference is; when uncle Tom (as he likes to be called) is in, there has been reports that Sweet-Potato is not touching her food and seems to be in discomfort but she drinks well. Staff has noticed this behaviour and when they found out that Pauline does not take a No for an answer and Sweet-P is scared of Pauline they tried to manipulate the situation when they were supporting her with nutritional needs e.g. "Sweet-potato, if you do not eat your food, I will call Pauline." Sweet-Potato will gradually take some of the food being offered. She is playing us up, you see, one of the carers commented. This trick is working, I will hand it over to the next coming shift, she continued. A few days later when

Sweet Potato was examined by her own General Physician, he found out that she has a defected tooth and swollen gums and was referred to the local dentist for further investigations and treatment. That summed up the reason for her declining to eat and preferring to drink only, she was suffering with pains and discomfort. An opportunity missed to relieve the service user's suffering and let her live a very pleasant life, enjoy her food and maintain her usual normal weight. This is just a tip of the ice bag.

"This is your fault that your family is not visiting you, you always complain and never get happy."

"Oh, we had a wonderful weekend, we went to the pier in Weston Super Mare", said Lulu to Virginia. Where?, asked the service user. Don't be nosy, we are not talking to you, and they both continued with their conversation, whilst attending to her personal care.

"No, no, no. we are definitely not taking Cindy out to the town centre, she always asks to be taken to the toilet every ten minutes".

"This is not you talking, Love; it is your dementia."

"Hello, hello, can someone help me please? (The voice continued, becoming more and more desperate with every minute passing by). In a minute, sounded the voice of a carer from a distance (rather very casual with no commitment)."

Again, person-hood undermined, person centre care approach dismantled. The challenges for carers and nurses are mounting and they are as steep as a hill they have never climbed before. Dementia is a challenge and every dementia sufferer is unique.

Social Changes in Life

Not only the psychological context is challenged to the dementia sufferers, but they find their social context way out of their control or shall I say, in the second hands. By the time they realise that they are moving backwards, not able to meet their friends, colleagues and go to their usual spots, enjoying shopping with family and / or friends they find themselves living on someone's schedule. Everything becomes distasteful. They are just shadows of themselves. Their movements are guided by laws and regulations. They are no longer free as birds. They choose what is originally not their choice. Needless to say their concerns might be viewed as argumentative and senseless and never followed up, never fully addressed or investigated. As Kitwood (2005) would say, personhood is undermined.

This is a depressing thought and damaging the self-esteem and self-worth. Look at this giant of a gentleman: Professor Nesta found himself reduced from a highly qualified academic, responsible father of two successful grown up sons, an enthusiastic sportsman (golfer), devoted Christian to a dependent dementia sufferer. He has been an intellectual with his own fruitful, rich lifestyle; having breakfast of choice at 07h30 (thanks to Olga, his faithful wife of 60 years); a visit to the shower room (he hated a bath – he fell when he was 10 years old and nearly broke his right ankle); choosing a decent outfit for the day to impress Olga and her possible competitors; plunging that, "I can't wait to see you again kiss", to his wife; and off to work with his sport car. He lived a dream life.

The only diary he needed to worry about being his and Olga's, for possible clashes with the work schedule, which will be rescheduled amicably and with a smile.

Then…

BOOM! The unexpected.

.The only way was not Essex, but straight to a care home as Olga proved to be too frail and too depressed to cope with the situation. Things became worse as the children were too far and could not help with the situation due to work schedules and child care commitments. That was the reverse of the fortunes as decisions had to be made for him.

If we stay close to mundane reality and explore how people with dementia live out their lives from day to day in their own homes and in the settings where formal care is provided, we get a very different picture. (Kitwood, 2005).

He further states that, "it is clear that many social or societal factors are involved: culture, locality, social class, education, financial resources, the availability or absence of support and services."

In fairness, some homes bring the social events in, so that people can feel at home, feel cared for and can enjoy themselves with their families and bond with staff members and other service users.

The Model – The Changing Times

The emergence of privately owned care sectors, residential and nursing care homes changed the care settings to different twists and turns. With changing times, demands, economic ups and downs, changing regulations, amendments in laws, new legislations and business gains and/or losses.

The business culture of care sector has changed the look and the focus into profit versus care. The biggest losers here are the service users and to a lesser extent the providers of care. The rising cost of care and the growing demand and changes in legislation has been an enormous factor that puts pressure on both families and care providers.

Sounds Familiar?

> "We are not allowed to use agency staff"
> -Management
> "For £6.00 an hour, I am not killing myself"
> -Care Staff
> "Are you short staffed again?"
> -Service User

These are just the drop in the ocean and sums up the rough road to the high quality of care.

It's not all doomed though, bravo to all those that have an outstanding rating from Care Quality Commission (CQC).

The magnitude of problems in care sectors is never in decline at the moment. Pressure is mounting from all angles.

Chapter One
"I am Scared"

"SOS!!! Fright is a Heavy Freight to Handle."

"I am scared," an eighty-eight-year-old lady said, shaking. I leaned forward and softly asked her, what are you afraid of? You people and this place, replied the old lady. I took a step backwards, maintaining the eye contact. She continued, I should not be afraid, but I know there is something wrong with me. What is wrong with you? I chipped in? I really don't know, she said. She looked at me and I noticed that she was really not comfortable at all. Let's finish the drink, I said, trying to distract her. Oh yeah, she said, a glimmer of joy sparked on her face as she pulled the beaker towards her mouth.

This is no gimmicks. Fright is the last thing that you can wish to have at any time in your lifetime, it paralyses you, it makes you feel helpless, empty and trapped. Living in fear can ruin your life. People underestimate fear and the challenges it comes out with.

The fear factor comes into place long before the resident is introduced to the care. It creeps in when the family and/or the resident identify the early warning signs of dementia. When families and friends are concerned about the ill-behaviour of their loved one's confusion, incontinent of both urine and faeces, forgetfulness, loss of interest, swearing and using very foul language when he/she has never done it before in his/her entire life this escalates worries and fears.

The fear of unknown, forgetting, confusion, loss of memory, poor judgement, loss of initiative, getting lost and wandering, loss of individuality (catching up with the activities of daily living – finances, preparing own meals and taking himself/herself to bed).

Christine Bryden, (2005) explains the experience as "changing as a person, losing the super-fast, super-smart me". She further notes that she slowed down and the world was becoming too fast for her. She was obviously losing touch with reality. When you reach that stage of dysfunction, not able to drive, not able to answer phones- that's very scary.

The dysfunction becomes worse for other people affected by dementia as they cannot even dress/undress themselves, develop hallucinations, suspicious behaviour (more common being refusing to eat because he/she thinks someone is trying to poison him/her and/or accusing people of hiding his /her belongings, etc.) The worst nightmare is when someone does not recognise his/her family members or when he/she is harmful to others and himself, for example, forgetting to turn off the gas or wanders off at night.

Families and their loved ones admitted in care homes can be scared for various reasons.

Their concern at the moment is how their loved ones will cope with the situation and how they (families) are going to cope with their loss. Care homes have proven to have a bad reputation in the past. People thought an elderly person is sent to care homes to die as one carer joked, "They are waiting for God."

Openness

Dementia is not an open and shut ordeal. We must allow people to talk openly about the disease. It is seen as a shameful, unwanted disease. Talking about it can ease the fear and pain/ suffering and encourage people to move forward or be keen to deal with dementia as early as they can. Bryden (2003), calls the experience of having dementia a "pit of despair". I think the longer the people looking after people who have been diagnosed with dementia fear and shy away from seeking help, the deeper this pit becomes and the more the disease engulfs the sufferer.

There is no comfort in being diagnosed with a disease that will totally change your life for good. Dementia is unlike other controllable diseases like diabetes mellitus or hypertension or hypotension, hyper/hypothyroidism, etc. It is not about watching your diet and keeping healthy habits. The road is on a downward spiral as the confusion, forgetfulness, etc. is rather deteriorating at an alarming rate. It is a slow walk to the unknown, fearful and not to mention the most dreadful experience.

People looking after dementia sufferers takes a back sit and leave it to the professionals to inject that key information in breaking the ice, that things won't be the same. Wisely enough, the professional approach is required and more suitable in the early stages as both parties are very vulnerable. This on its own is not enough. It needs to be continuously followed by small talks with the person suffering from dementia and the rest of other family members.

Below here Bear's story explains why we should not underestimate people suffering from dementia as their fear of dementia can turn our lives upside down as well, if we do not deal with the situation openly and fairly.

I had just reported for duty when a carer rushed to the equipment room and came out with a wheelchair at 15 if not 20mph. Hey, what's going on?, I asked. You are going to run someone down if you are not careful, I carried on. We have an emergency, she exploded.

One of the new residents went out through the patio door and is refusing to come back in and says he is going home. I put my belongings behind the desk and followed her. There was a crew outside surrounding the resident. They managed to encourage him to get inside the building. This was not an easy task by any means. As they approached the entrance he promised them that if they did not allow him to talk to his wife, he is going to smash everything made from glass in the building. He sounded and looked very serious and by his looks he meant every vowel and consonant he muttered.

He looked at every one of us as if he is studying us and asked, "do I look mental to you?" You look very upset at the moment Sir, replied one of the member of staff (nice swerve – I said to myself). Bear, please, he smiled at the staff showing them he was comfortable when called by his first name. This is a mental institution, am I right? Bear continued to poke with his questions. Yes and no, Bear. This is a home which looks after the elderly, including dementia and we also accept respite clients. I see, Bear nodded.

"Not my wife, my wife will never do that to me," he added. It's Jade, my daughter in law.

Why is she doing this to me? I know it's her, she wanted to get rid of me for a long time. She is so cruel, so mean.

It was about time to take Jade out of the picture as the mention of her name fuels more anger towards Bear and huge fear towards staff and other residents. Fortunately, her wife rang and was informed about the situation and allowed her to speak to him not for long, as the conversation was more confrontational and moving back to Jade. Bear's argument was the fact that he was not involved in this decision. He felt bullied by one of the family members as he believed that his sons and wife did not make the final decision.

He was willing to sit down with his family and discuss this situation. He felt every move was done behind his back. We managed to encourage him to go to bed and revisit the situation in the morning when all the family and management are in the building. He managed to settle and promised that he was not going to cause any problems.

Snow-Pot Effect

We somewhat fail to understand the difficulties physically, emotionally, spiritually and otherwise that these people are undergoing. There is nothing devastating and upsetting when you feel you are not understood and you have nowhere to go. The words, I understand, has been reassured, do not worry, does not entirely take the problem away. What we should understand is the fact that by the time we meet them in our institutions, these problems are at the peak of their levels. They might not have been necessary, dealt with at this stage, but they might have caused a tremendous damage to our clients, it might be months or years, who knows?

People react differently to even similar situations. Life is unpredictable and to some extent very complicated, it's not as simple as we might think.

Below is a graph that shows how fear engulfs our clients and families. This list is neither exhaustive nor rigid by any means.

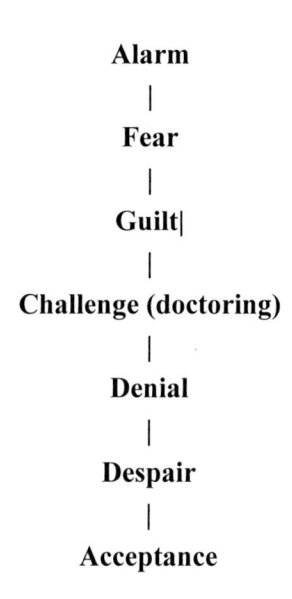

Alarm
|
Fear
|
Guilt|
|
Challenge (doctoring)
|
Denial
|
Despair
|
Acceptance

This is called the snow-pot-effect. There is a lot of input and twists and turns resulting in one solution, be it to institutionalise, or look after the sufferer at home in this case. There are mixed feelings, but they bring about unity. The results are clear and decisions are final and mostly not regrettable.

Alarm

When the alarm bell rings, everything comes to a standstill, there are showers of doubts and disbelief. Who does not want to turn the alarm off when he/she is not ready to wake up? "What are we going to do now?" the confusion, indecisiveness, doubts, sympathy, sadness, astonishment and disbelief clouds the families. This might not be new to the observer, but there is really no time for "what if's". One needs to act fast as soon as possible before the situation gets out of hands. Everybody is running around looking for answers to their questions. It is the day of confusion, headaches and loads of consultations.

Fear

This is the worst feeling everybody dreads. Fear of being told you have dementia or your loved one has dementia is the worst nightmare. You really do not know where to start or what to believe. "Do we spread the news or not?", "What if we are wrong?", "How are we going to deal with this?", "Are we really losing our parent/ brother/sister?". The grip of fear is immense.

Guilt

That feeling of guilt creeps in and people start wondering if it's their fault and could they have done something different to prevent this from occurring. "We have failed him/her", self-blames continues. You have that urge to do something, maybe it's not too late. At this time life trends into memorable flashes. Something has changed, life is not the same. "I do",

"Till death do us apart" seems distant; "in sickness and in health" seems doubtable.

Challenge

There is a growing confidence and determination. We can dot these i's and cross these t's is the spirit. Hopes of "I wish this will go away", "We can turn this around", "this is just temporary", "he/she will pull through", "it's not too late to act" encourages people to shop around (doctor shopping) for advice, treatments, diagnosis (hoping for anything but not dementia). The reality and the permanence of the disease has not sunk in. There is still hope-false hope and the time is running out. The strength and the enduring powers and spirit of the family is being tested to the limit. The race is on for the solution to this predicament.

Denial

The disbelief, fear of the unknown grows day by day. Dementia changes people's lives for good. This is an unbearable loss. This is not what families want to hear. "This is not happening", "There must be a mistake", "It can't be my father/mother", are the daily echoes. The action that follows delays early diagnosis and treatment and better preparations of the entire family, including the sufferer to deal with the disease.

Despair

It's like watching a very exciting, nice movie and suddenly whilst enjoying it the curtains are drawn and there's a big sign, THE END. But this time the difference is, it's gone forever, there is no repeat or revisit. That was the last, live picture.

Acceptance

This is by no means the easiest decision. It is a very bitter pill to swallow. It is like accepting a familiar stranger in your house and locked in for the rest of your life. It is the start of a new, unfamiliar journey as every routine will change irrespective of keeping your loved one at home or taking him/her to a care home. It is a challenge and needs bravery. "Dementia was a shameful disease, to be feared or denied not one to be acknowledged and battled with", as Bryden (2005), claims.

Chapter Two
"Where Is You Born?"

It was just after lunch, twenty three minutes to two to be precise. The sun shone through the big floral curtained windows. The lounge was full of residents, some dozing off, some busy with activities and some chatting with their loved ones. It was quiet, you could hear the shuffling of the playing cards and the soft snoring of some residents who declined to go to their bedrooms for an afternoon snooze and stretched themselves in their comfortable reclining chairs and then…the sound exploded from the far end.

"Where is you born?" asked the carer in a rather loud and alarming voice. Suddenly everything went dead quiet, the new resident looked very astonished, with questioning, appealing eyes.

"Where is who?" asked the resident. "You born?" repeated the carer. I don't know who you are talking about, whoever he or she is I don't know, never mind her whereabouts, replied the resident, showing signs of anxiety now. "Are you wearing your hearing aid?" she asked, pointing to her ears. No, I do not have hearing aid, I can still hear perfectly well my darling, you don't have to shout. Okay, let's start again, the carer continued. Where is you born? for instance in London, Swindon or here in Northampton.

Oh! Is that what you meant, I am a Londoner, she boastedly replied.

It all dawned on us that she meant, "Where were you born?" That's communication for you, you miss one thing the whole context is gone astray and you start to blame the other party for misunderstanding you. Communication when dealing with people with dementia is a key starting from stage one to end of life. We are quick at jumping to conclusion that, oh! They are confused whilst we put them at that state of confusion sometimes.

Dementia clients are well known to lose their concentration easily, lapse in memory, irritability, anxiety etc.

B. MacCarthy (2011) explains why communication when it comes to dementia to be specific is a real disturbing struggle. "We communicate to get a message across the others to share ideas with others and to find out what others think and feel, to build intimacy, to share and solve problems." He goes on, "Without the ability to communicate we struggle to maintain a source of relationship, connection and psychological attachment to people."

The struggle with communication should by all means not be a two way process. The preparedness of caregivers to be one or two steps ahead of the service users should be standard. There is no way that institutions can curb the problems affecting the service users if they do not step up one level to improve poor communication. Training on different aspects of care, skills including communication skills with special emphasis on dementia, understanding the ups and downs of living with dementia, family support etc., is of vital importance. The connection and understanding between the communicating parties gives positive re-enforcement, that feeling of togetherness, the zest for happiness, that "when will I see you again (tantalizing smile)".

How many times have we heard people saying, oh! Mary (resident) loves Jane (carer).

One will ask, what is Jane doing that the other carers cannot do? Although this promotes favouritism, it sometimes works especially when we all chip in with a good work, care and love to fill the gap nicely and ensure you all care and good as Jane. What makes residents feel at home when she is on should be a common practice for all given that the homes are promoting team work and person centred care and all should follow what Jane does well, if it's legal of course.

Handovers, sharing of ideas, care plan reviews, client conferencing, do iron out these niggling concerns.

Time is money, under done it could be a loss, over done it could be costly. Every second wasted in care count polish your communication skills. The balance is key. People react differently to same situations or same to different situations.

This is far from easy, understandable but not excusable. We do not have enough staff and / or we don't have time to say the least, can be dealt with.

Better still, one thing leads to another. Two wrongs don't produce the right thing, but two wrongs can be turned into the right direction and produce good to better results. The good example is the introduction of care certificates in the care sector. Cavendish Review (2013) likened care as a disconnected landscape, "I have been struck by how disconnected the systems are which care for the public. The National Health Services (NHS) operates in silos, and social care is seen as distant land occupied by a different tribe." It also found out that training and development of healthcare assistants and adult social care workers were often not consistent or good enough. The review recommended a rigorous quality assurance for training courses and vocational qualifications. Cavendish proposed that a new "Certificate of Fundamental Care" be created to improve this and this resulted in "Care Certificate".

The care certificates cover the learning outcomes, competencies and standards of behaviours that must be expected. There are about 15 Standards that make up the certificate. These form the integral part of care. Every care assistant who has undergone thorough training and has passed and obtained the care certificate and determined and dedicated to care, will be as good as gold.

The certificate touches in detail every aspect of care from the initial stages including communication, personal care, moving and handling, challenging behaviours, care planning, risk assessments and risk management, palliative care etc. Some institutions have introduced the care certificate as standard. This has proved to be the best move as the new ones are empowered at the earliest stages of their careers with knowledge, skills, awareness and preparedness to tackle any problems coming their way.

Chapter Three

"Do you think it's funny that people don't care what's going to happen to you?"

How many times do we hear the cries, "I have been dumped, no one cares about me."

Betty was sitting on her armchair facing the window and her back was towards the door of her bedroom. It was dark in her bedroom (her choice obviously as when she heard the footsteps, she shouted -whoever you are and whatever you are doing leave the lights off please). That was more than enough to enforce silence in the room and then she turned around, eyes pinpointed at me. She looked very concern. With a rather disturbed voice she said, "Do you think it's funny that people don't care what's going to happen to you?"

Interestingly the whole cabinet was full of family photos, young and matured. There was one that caught my eye, it was placed forward and distanced from others. Who is this handsome man? I asked. He is the reason why I am here and now he is selling my house because he cannot do what I did to him, caring for him until he was a grown up man. Oh, that must be the son, I muttered to myself. Anger was written all over her face and there was no way at that moment I could calm her down other than to give her space, obviously reassuring her that we do care and treat everyone with respect and dignity.

Being away from your loved ones is a bitter pill to swallow. In fact the most disturbing and frustrating thing is when you are trying to ponder why are you in an institution and someone else is carelessly telling you, "This is your home now love". Which is by the way very much true, but, is the timing right? Is the message conveyed in the right manner? Does he/she feel at home? Destiny still eludes us. Is it end to the means or the means to the end? In a very normal circumstances we become masters of our own destiny, be it pleasurable or otherwise but in dementia it's a different ball game.

Why the behavioural change? Early stages of admission are the most crucial. The early painful divorce from your loved ones is unbearable. That feeling of emptiness, loneliness, sadness, and tearfulness is heart-breaking.

Let's not forget the heartache goes both ways. When families are faced with such a big decision to make, where there is no other option but to move their loved ones to the nursing home, it is undeniable the painful experience to endure. We do know how the residents feel, taking from what we see and what we hear and what we observe during their stay, but what the families do experience is still a mystery as they try to battle with their loss. We don't know what happens in those closed doors. We don't witness those broken hearts and those tears-soaked pillows and those guilty feelings. That brave outlook contrasted with that broken heart and soul is astonishingly unbelievable.

Nursing homes are the last resort after all avenues have been exhausted. As noted in chapter one, dementia is the most dreaded disease in the whole world and it's growing rapidly. Families are the weakest link, not in terms of their contribution or part they take but their reluctance to break the ice and deal with the diagnosis at the earliest stages, refer immediately they notice and suspect symptoms and accept treatment. They fear the future because nursing homes are associated with poor care, neglect and death. By the time they bring their loved ones to the nursing home after all the efforts you can see the despair in their eyes and you can read, "THIS IS IT", clearly written in their eyeballs. Very few approach the moving in as a rehabilitative attempt. Some start distancing themselves, not that they do not want to be part of the process but the loss is unbearable.

To see his/her colleagues and/or friends living their lives to the fullest, to see her/him trying to cope with the new routine and lost in thoughts, asking unanswered questions- whys and hows.

Pre-admission taster works sometimes, where a prospective client is introduced to the home, spend some time with staff and other residents to see if he/she would like the place. The taster helps the client to explore options, maximize choices and have questions asked and answered. This introductory phase is very important as the engagement between the families, clients and staff and clients/client interaction is put to the test and ties may be strengthened. It allows openness, sharing of achievements and increases trust.

This can be a vital moment for the nursing home staff to invite a specialist dementia person to answer all concerns and myths about dementia.

Chapter Four

"Can I please go and spend a penny?"

The call-bell rang and Mary-Ann jumped to attend the caller. Who is it Mary? Mary-Ann not Mary, she exploded. Can you answer the question whoever you are, please, pleaded John sluggishly. The new lady in room 1603. Does she have a name? That's not funny John, she continued her walk to room 1603. She did not take much time and she came back and sat quietly on the armchair. We waited and Mary-Ann surprisingly said nothing. We looked at each other and then we almost asked her simultaneously, but the nurse beat us to it. Anything to report Mary-Ann?, asked the nurse. Oh, I just told her to try and get some sleep. Why was she ringing the bell, Mary-Ann?, continued the nurse. She said she wants to spend a penny. You tell me, which shop is open after midnight.

Imagine taking her on a wheelchair down the road at this time, she continued with a very sarcastic giggle and shrugging her shoulders. She had a very confident smile and full of herself until… "Mary-Ann can we have a word please, in the office and you two can you please attend to Jane (the service user)", said the nurse very concerned and rather astonished by Mary-Ann's reaction.

When nature calls, there's neither ifs nor buts, there's no "in a minute" (which in some care homes is equivalent to up to half an hour or indefinite). When you need to go, you must go. It is as simple as that. Residents are made to wait for a very uncomfortable period before they are being attended to. That's an undeniable, sad, embarrassing fact.

It is such a shame when a place called home does not understand your basic needs. Is it lack of cultural understanding / knowledge? This can create serious problems when residents revert to slang and/or other forms of communicating that the person caring for her/him is not familiar with. Caring is not as easy as one might think. The key is to ask when you do not understand. Do not assume. No one is perfect, better be safe than sorry.

There are a whole lot of challenges and barriers to come across. Culture plays a big role in our lives. There is an old saying that, when in Rome, do as the Romans do. This is no coincidence to caring, when you come in the world of dementia be smart and ready.

Whatever you get yourself into, first dangle your feet in and get used to the temperature.

Never run too fast and never walk too fast either. Enjoy the ride, learn every mile and count every minute passing by because dementia is a very challenging interesting disease.

Mixing

Ignorance is no excuse in dealing with dementia, but there might be tiny things that could surprise us. We learn almost every day. "I am Irish and I drink tea with milk and not milk with tea". That was well said by Yvonne. It needed no repetition and needed no interpretation as well. I felt I have been "read the riot act". I was shell shocked as I thought I was not doing anything wrong. I apologised sincerely.

Yvonne might have been watching me when I was doing the tea round, I assume. Preparing her tea, I assembled her cup and saucer and asked her how many sugars does she take (Note, I did not say how much sugar does she take). She replied, tea, milk and no sugar. I poured milk from the milk jug, followed by the tea from the tea-pot, then… the hell broke loose. I immediately made a fresh cup and it was received with a smile. I thanked her for teaching me Irish culture and promised her that I will be coming for more tips.

That's the beauty of culture. If we do not dig deep and learn more about the residents we are looking after, we might be caught napping and that can grossly affect our care. The more we familiarise ourselves with the culture of our clients, the better we get into grips with their needs, good to best care planning, clear historical background and better understanding of our clients. Health professionals, care assistants, care givers and other related disciplines need to be clear about the cultural issues.

We are all influenced by our cultural background, what we have learnt when we grew up. A person's identity is also shaped amongst other things by their own personality, education, family experience, socioeconomic status and life experiences. When looking at the field of dementia, one way of incorporating a person's cultural background is through the concept of person-centred care. With this approach, you can treat each person as an individual and consider all aspects of the person's background. (Cited from Dementia Training Study Centre – An Australian Government Initiative).

There is still a growing concern about the impact of culture and language in care. Tom Kitwood (2005) said, "If there are such powerful forces to preserve the status quo and to sabotage the beginnings of positive change, we might well ask how a new culture of dementia care could possibly come into being. It will not happen through a paradigm shift that is merely at the level of theory."

Cultural and language differences is where the problems start and escalates in care. This leads to misunderstandings, frustrations, fear of being neglected and not cared for. This can bring about a feeling of dejection and challenging behaviour. Care can be compromised, residents can be offered what they did not wish for, care not up to their required standard and this can bring the home into disrepute. The importance of inclusion of family and a translator at the earliest stages is very vital as some concerns can be ironed out.

The other interesting thing about the elderly is the fact that some revert to their original mother tongue at the later stages. This makes matters even more worse, a nightmare for the caring staff. This comes as a surprise to the staff, especially when you come one morning and the resident you used to get along fine with does no longer speak the same language as you are.

Just imagine the Bulgarian example I cited in chapter 2, attending to a client who only communicate using nonverbal cues. Just a simple thing, a menu. When offered a choice, Menu A and B, the resident may shake his/her head on the first preference A and nod on B or vice-versa. For someone who understands differently this is not a clear-cut decision. The staff attending to this resident may end up making a wrong decision and the resident may be the one at the receiving end, at the end of the day.

These are the niggling problems which should be tackled earlier on when planning, admission, not when the problem has already escalated. We should be planning ahead and get our plans implemented and our resources made available when needed.

Chapter Five

"She must be blonde, eh."

Bravo blondes, bravo! I think they have reigned for decades. Who said sexuality has no room in the elderly? Wow, life is amazing.

Hello smiler, she said, leaning forward on her bed with a broad smile, waving vigorously with her right hand. Hi Geraldine, how are you today? Nice to see you smiler, I am so glad to see you, she holds her fists together and punched the air, giggling. It was like we have not seen each other for weeks and yet it was the previous night when we met for the first time. I might have done a good job on my previous shift, I muttered to myself. I wish she was my boss (it's very hard to please those species), I continued with my duties.

The tantalizing fairy-tale went on. It was about four weeks when I was assigned duties at where Geraldine was. As I was about to attend to her, another service user living adjacent to her room rang the call-bell for assistance. Can someone help me please? She went on.

She sounded distressed and was crying, oh, oh, please! I rushed off quickly, fearing the worst. Margaret, hello, what's the matter? How can I be of help? I asked a bit concerned. I looked around and by mere glance she was not in any physical danger. I have just tucked myself in and realised that my drinks table is far. Margaret, I have just called the whole defence force and the emergency services, thinking that you are in great danger, I said joking. No, you did not, she replied, eyes wide open. Oh, come on Margaret you can reach this, I said jokingly as the table was about one and a half meters away from her. We both laughed it off and I said, good night Margaret and she replied, same to you. I proceeded to Geraldine, right where were we? My chatty old lady was a bit quiet and she looked at me and said, you never laughed like that with me, "she must be blonde, eh". I was lost for words and reassured her that she will always get attention from staff members.

Residents, both genders have liberty to make their choices, be it fairy tales or temporary adjustments to their lives or a stop to what was an enjoyable journey.

Where Do We Stand?

Below are the two selected scenarios:

Jasmine was admitted in a care home looking after people with dementia. She was married to a gentleman called John. Jasmine had children of her own, two daughters she was fond of and John had only one son who was overseas, a thousand miles away. They have been married for twenty seven years, led a very good life and John loved the girls as if they were his own. They have been a close-knit family.

John did not take long to follow Jasmine as he was admitted in the same care home with Alzheimer's disease. They were placed in the double room and were sharing all facilities. This was a lovely re-union and both were happy about it. Jasmine deteriorated rapidly and was more confused and disorientated. John had more insight than Jasmine. At this point they were still aware that they are husband and wife, but the confusion outweighed any fruitful conversation or attachment. They will kiss each other good night at bedtime though (they never miss this part).

The conversation became more irrelevant at times. They were in separate beds, but from time-to-time staff looking after them during the night found John next to Jas's bed and his excuse always was, "I want to ensure she is warm enough". Jas complained to her daughters saying he is hurting her. There was little evidence to support that statement as Jas was confused and keep changing her statement, but the family decided to separate them as they said he is distressing their mother. John was placed in another care home away from Jasmine. That's the family torn apart.

Scenario 2

Jolene met Peter in the care home (both widowed). They became close friends when they met in the home's activities, competing in quiz shows, active in games, brilliant in gardening and participating in home chores. They started spending time together in lounges, dining halls and on home trips. Both families accepted their friendship which grew even closer and faster than the people thought. This was a fairy tale, a sweet unchained melody. They respected each other, respected the staff and everybody liked them. They were a very decent couple, they were whole again.

When emotions run very high, decisions can be more harmful than good. We tend to forget to value their choices and absolutely not thinking in their context. We rip off their reasoning and give them no opportunity to stand for themselves. And yet again the balance of our scales is lopsided.

Let us not forget that our positive contribution is not judged by how we stand alongside the strong but how we stand strong for the weakest. People affected by dementia lose their identity and self-worth.

Inconsistency

Let us look at Mrs D's story.

Mrs D, a no-nonsense woman in her late 80's used to tell all the staff that, "the only man who entered my bedroom was my husband." That was loud and crystal clear – she did not want to be attended to by a male care staff, especially personal care.

This was respected and valued by the staff and was documented. This was becoming very tricky with staff shortage as the home will cover with agency workers and often male carers will be sent. Staff would try their "luck" and try to overturn that preference but the iron lady stood firm.

Unfortunately, as the disease progressed she deteriorated and at the end of life stage, when the energy levels were down, limbs given up, eyes could not give that, "you dare not", stare, voiceless, that privacy and dignity went through the window. Her wishes and preferences were just on a paper as she was attended by male carers in confusion. What a pity?

Dementia sufferers are entitled to be respected and valued irrespective of cognitive impairment. They do not deserve to have little joy followed by torment when they least expect to die happily with dignity.

Chapter Six

"It's your dementia, love."

Adam rang the call bell and was pacing up and down in his room. When the carer came in to attend to him, he slowly went to sit down on his armchair. He sighed and clutched his head with both arms and said, tell me it was just a dream. He looked very distraught.

Without even looking at him the carer who came to attend to his needs, wrapped it up, try to sleep, "it's your dementia, love". Why did he ring the call-bell? What was this dream about? Why did he look so distraught? These questions remained unanswered. Alzheimer's disease and other dementia sometimes cause people to behave in ways that are different and difficult for others to live with, for example, people with dementia may become restless or aggressive for no obvious reason. (Bailey, p98)

How many times have we heard that? Oh! It's Jane, she is playing up again. Most people who have or are looking after people with dementia sometimes felt that they are being taken for a ride or that the other person is being deliberately mischievous.

People with dementia often do child-like things or may just appear bewildered or perplexed at times. This is the result of the illness. It is not a deliberate attempt to annoy.

(Bailey, p99)

Across the United Kingdom, most health care institutions have embarked on various projects and intensive training on dementia awareness, respect and dignity. Are we doing enough?

Is labelling accepted for some and a taboo for some? Is it because they are so defenceless, we can pick and choose what we call them? Do we have to remind them of their plight?

Dementia affects people in different ways. As it has been mentioned before, people with dementia react differently to the same situations or same to different situations.

Lumping people together under the label of dementia and approaching them, in the same way, is likely to increase problems of communication and make it difficult for us to hear their voice. (Goldsmith, p35)

People with dementia forget things, sees things, remember some things, misplaces things, hear things and have their way of dealing with the things. Dementia presents itself in different astonishing ways. Observe, listen, interact, reassure and consult.

Types of Dementia

The most common types of dementia with courtesy of the leaders in dementia research, training, care and treatment, the Alzheimer's Society are: Alzheimer's, Vascular Dementia, Lewy's body Dementia and Fronto temporal Dementia amongst the list. As it has been mentioned before, there are different types of dementia affecting people in different ways and people behaving in different ways.

The word Dementia is an umbrella encompassing different behaviours and those should not be blanketed when dealing with a person with dementia.

Alzheimer's disease

This is the most common cause of dementia. During the course of disease, the chemistry and structure of the brain changes leading to the death of brain cells.

Vascular Dementia

If the oxygen supply to the brain fails, brain cells may die. The symptoms of vascular dementia can either occur suddenly following a stroke or over time through a series of small strokes.

Dementia with Lewy's bodies

This form of dementia get its name from tiny spherical structures that develop inside the nerve cells. Their presence in the brain leads to the degeneration of brain tissue.

Frontotemporal dementia

In frontotemporal dementia, damage is usually found in the front part of the brain. Personality and behaviour are initially more affected than memory.

Creutzfeldt-Jakob disease (CJD)

This is the rare type of dementia and the most feared by families as it is associated with a short life-span when a person is affected by this type of dementia.

Prions are infectious agents that attack the central nervous system and then invade the brain causing dementia. The best-known prion is CJD.

Features

These are defining factors which can serve as guidelines to the care we give and can determine the planning of our care and relevant assessments. I think it is the duty of every person dealing with people affected by dementia to be aware of what he/she is dealing with. There is quite an overlap on some of the symptoms of these types of dementia, which explains the different behaviour and why people suffering from the disease should not be labelled as "one lot" but as individuals whose needs are being compromised and need help and support. These are some of the symptoms cited from the Alzheimer's Society.

Frontotemporal dementia

Features- Personality and behavioural changes, difficulty with language, loss of interest in people and things, lose sympathy and/or empathy, show compulsive behaviour, hoarding and obsessed with time-keeping, impaired understanding of complex sentences, but not single words, slow hesitant speech and errors in grammar e.g., leaving small links like "to", "from" or "the".

Vascular Dementia

Features- problems with planning and organizing, a slower speed of thought, lack of concentration, problems recalling recent events. Problems perceiving objects in three dimensions, mentally and socially active, more common in men than women, it has even double the risk with people having stroke, diabetes and hypertension.

Alzheimer's disease

Features-memory lapses, difficulty recalling recent events and learning new information, lose items, forget recent events, get lost in familiar places, forget appointments/anniversaries, concentration, planning and organizing affected, challenging behaviour at a later stage, eating and mobility problems.

Lewy's bodies

Features-depression, visual hallucinations, delusions, Parkinson's disease like symptoms, mobility problems- shuffling and trembling, speech and swallowing difficulties.

Creutzfeldt-Jakob's disease

Features- progresses within six months, loss of interest, jerky movements, shakiness, stiffness of limbs, continence, loss of ability to move or speak and unaware of surroundings.

Knowledge is power. Such knowledge can be abused as easily as it can be used positively. It can be used to manipulate other people to do things, or stop doing things without them being aware of what is happening. Apparently, innocent words like "influence", "persuasion" and even "encouragement" might be hiding a degree of covert behaviour and coercion designed to disguise the motivation behind the intervention. "Henderson and Atkins, 2003"

They further argue that first they have the power and secondly many of the people who use their services are vulnerable. The combination of power and vulnerability creates all the ingredients for the potential abuse of knowledge of human behaviour.

Chapter Seven

"The word you are looking for is bored, bored and bored to the bone."

Where's everybody gone? She was sitting in a small lounge. Sadly all the other residents vacated the lounge and went to their bedrooms. She was in no hurry to go anywhere but seemed queeringly surprised. Television was off. Clutching her handbag with her left arm, she asked if she can have a cup of coffee. Certainly, I said and went straight to the mini kitchen and prepared a cup of coffee for her and offered her. As I put the cup in front of her, she looked at me and asked, is it your first time here? Yes, I said.

When a service user complains about boredom, then there is a cause for concern. We might look at it both ways – we offered, she refused, she is a woman of her own word, she is untouchable, she was occupied with family, she was asleep, she had an appointment, she was not very well, she was not in a good mood, she is sometimes confused and forgets.

The first initial stages of admission are the most crucial to get the service users engaged in home activities and routine. Let them settle, do not bombard them with lots of responsibility and commitments – this is kind of tricky and difficult. Residents are not the same. They may share the same diagnosis but reacts differently and needs to be treated individually. Given the fact that some symptoms ranges from loss of interest, problems with language, socially detached, lack of understanding complex tasks and semantic at times, we really have a mountain to climb. Taking a trip down memory lane does not take a red London bus to do. It needs skills, patience, perseverance, understanding and empathy.

"Research has shown that mice with dementia kept in an enriched environment where they are stimulated both mentally and physically can learn new tasks, remember old ones and develop new brain cells. Yet every nursing home she saw, stacked their inmates around a room with a television blaring in the middle. No one was encouraged to talk, exercise or even walk. Life in a nursing home slowly, inexorably dehumanizes its resident." (Cited in Whitman (2010), p131-132)

There are currently many articles and views about activities and older people. In the past years research has shown that activities play a large part in preventing the progression of dementia. It is also known that socializing prevents loneliness, despair and suicidal thoughts. (Cited from National Association for Providers of Activities for Older People (2005, p24).

Meaningful activities are essential or shall I say a must for maintaining physical and psychological wellbeing. Older people who disengage from activity through illness, disability or social isolation experience diminished health and wellbeing. Meaningful activity may be used therapeutically as an agent for a positive change.

Generalized activities are not always fruitful but the past/present history is more appropriate and maybe well received. People change. What they used to like and enjoy may not be their cup of tea and what they are taught in later life may be far from their liking. They say never teach an old dog new tricks. According to Jean Carper, (2010, p147) physical inactivity makes an individual a more attractive target for memory loss and Alzheimer's disease.

Keep it simple but not ridiculous. Remember you might be dealing with academics who will not be pleased when their intellectual capabilities are challenged/ undermined.

Communicate your plans across, agree and stick to the agreed terms and bear in mind you are not dealing with dementia but with people affected by dementia.

The Lost Treasure

He was 80 years old, she was 90 and a half. Good innings and they were still on the pitch. She had mental capacity, and so did he. She was a fighter, he was a peacemaker. She was bit of a stirrer sometimes, he was nice but not a pushover. She can talk for hours but he still had that courage to listen to her and drift to sleep when he is tired.

Renee, what can I do, please help me, said Bee sounding a bit distressed. Me neither darling, I don't know what to do. I am just going to sit next to you now. Is it not that wonderful, just sitting down and do nothing, she continued. We are in the same boat, my love. It is like they said when we got married, together until death do us apart and in illness and health, I don't remember all that marriage rhyme but it's something like that. We used to have very interesting, enthusiastic ideas, competing, full of strength and now we are down to one called "nothing to do". We have seen the highs and lows of life. This is more than experience, this is wisdom. We are not as good as we used to be but we are ok.

Is that not bizarre? Welcome to old age my little boy, do not fight it, just accept it.

You know the funny thing about life, you have to adapt to the process of change. Make room for everything. Think where we were 50 years ago when we got married; going places, visiting friends and family members, playing with children and then came grandchildren. You were the best with children, I used to envy you because they all used to enjoy playing and talking to you. I love you, you have been a breath of fresh air in my life. We lived our lives to the fullest, I have no regrets. We treasured every moment. Everything was looking rosy. That is all gone now.

Teamwork is vital. Consultation is prime. Use every available relevant resource you have access to. Health care system has got links -physiotherapists, psychologists, social workers, doctors, specialists and psychiatrists, to name the few.

She goes on to say, "Generally, the more sedentary you are, the faster your cognitive decline." Researchers in the University of California, San Francisco found that older adults who were sedentary had the worst cognitive functioning at start of the seven-year study and the steepest decline throughout the study.

Activities should be person based if it's one to one and if it's a group a fair mix according to their background, understanding, age group, beliefs, orientation and capabilities. The activity must focus on stimulation of the individual/s rather than to occupy them. It must be tolerable, enjoyable, effective, uncomplicated and non-exhaustive. Do not go with the flow but encourage progress and also lift those who are struggling.

The process should be ongoing. Some homes have special weekend activities but some treat weekends as a family time giving opportunities for the working families who have limited time to visit their loved ones. The variety works. It reduces boredom and gives them something to think about. Variety, choice boosts confidence and increase that sense of belonging and self-worth and restore dignity. Bringing back those decision powers by letting them choose and have the final decision if it's appropriate.

Chapter Eight

"I am paying you."

Where does that come from? There is a saying in English that, there is no smoke without a fire. These are very strong words and when they are said they are thrown with a lot of vernon in heated situations. Usually, they are not welcome with positive responses, but if they are – well done you. Residents are paying for the services rendered to them and technically, the ugly truth is they are paying us. This is debatable.

Keep calm and care. Retaliating to the resident's anger is not the solution at this point as it aggravates matters. As it has been said before where there is smoke, there is fire. We are dealing with psychologically and physically traumatized individuals and as much as we detest that, we should handle them with care. This is a far cry for help, a cry for dissatisfaction on a greater scale a feeling of being misunderstood, unanswered questions very much overdue.

Residents are different but all are equal in the eyes of caring. Dealing with challenging behaviour can be very tricky. You can be dealing with a one-off situation where a resident is extremely annoyed/dissatisfied with issues of her own or care-related issues and after some time settles/calm down and often will apologise for the behaviour or forget the whole scenario.

Every behaviour has an explanation, it could be relevant or otherwise. Residents feel betrayed by the ones they love - family and by the ones they trust to look after them- care providers. The more the frustrations escalate, the more outbursts are witnessed. We may see these incidents as coming out of the blue but actually, they are triggered by the processes within the system.

They are on survival mode if I am allowed to put it that way. Being institutionalised is not their choice. The new adjustment to life is daunting. What they are experiencing is real in their context and how they deal with it is the correct way to them. They need to be understood and dealt with professionally. They have reached a degree of uncertainty and despair. They feel disempowered and believe they have the urge to fight back and regain their status. To be surrounded by strangers in a new unfamiliar environment is disturbing and absolutely, not homely especially when you have not settled. They have their rights scrapped without realising.

When care home residents realise that they are no longer a part of their human world, they experience despair. These feelings of such despair may be manifested through nonspecific complaints of physical or psychological distress and the resident may be stereotyped as hypochondria, mentally unstable, depressed or just a complainer. (RCN 1993)

People with dementia sometimes see things that other people cannot see. We might say they imagine things but to them, that is actually a reality.

Have you ever been punched and after realised that actually, it was your fault? It does happen. Hear my story with Jack (resident). It was early on a Sunday morning at the end of British winter/beginning of summer 2003. Jack likes to be up early, six o'clock to be exact, ready for breakfast, as the family will pick him up on Sunday to go to church. As we assisted him to bed I told him that I will be the one to assist him in the morning, will give him a shower and dress him. We said our good-nights and Jack retired to bed. He slept very well all night. He was up once when he went to the toilet (assisted to the commode by one carer) at around midnight.

Planning care for the morning, Jack was the first as agreed with him and his family. Jack is one of those people, if he said 6 o'clock he means at the dot not before and not after.

You do not want Jack to say you are early or late because that will be something that will echo in your ears for the whole week or two until he forgets that or decides not to pursue the matter. I timed myself and at exactly six o'clock I was on his bedside trying to get him up. Usually, when you agreed time with him, by that time he would be ready.

Jack was half- asleep and by no means ready to get up, which was strange (did I take notice of that? NO). Jack, it's time to get up, I said softly. No, he replied. Its six o'clock in the morning Jack. He looked at me and looked at the wall and looked away. I tapped him gently on his left shoulder and asked, are you not ready Jack? He turned and without any warning, BOOM! His right fist landed on my chest, missing my chin by an inch. I backed off and surprised, oh Jack that was not nice. What did you do that for? He did not answer back but looked at the wall and looked away. Alright then

Jack I will come back when you are ready, I said, very disappointed.

I really cannot believe this, I said to my colleagues, telling them what happened. He became very aggressive out of a blue, unpredictable, I continued. You must record that, said Roxie (the carer). I will definitely do an incident report, I replied. Ok, that's that let me carry on with my work and I will come back to Jack later. We will inform the family that he declined assistance at six o'clock if we run a bit late because of that incident. I will give him an hour and I will try again.

I went into the office to clear the night's work and update the administrative duties and went back to Jack, the time now was seven o'clock.

He was up, "the usual Jack". Hello Jack, I greeted him again. He smiled and said, good morning, with his deep voice. Are you ready now Jack? I asked. Oh, yeah, said Jack. I assisted him in the shower room. He enjoyed a luke-warm shower (as he like it). We spoke about the weather and the church service he was going to attend. After assisting him with dressing up he said he will prefer to wait in his room for breakfast and be ready when his son comes to fetch him for a church. We both agreed that was a good idea. He rested on his comfortable reclining chair. He said, thank you for helping me and I enjoyed the shower. You are welcome, Jack.

I decided to revisit the incident (obviously not happy about the incident), still thinking I did not do anything wrong to Jack and I did not deserve to be smacked. Jack, you hit me early in the morning. He replied, yeah (nodding) and I am very sorry for that. Why did you do that Jack?, I asked.

He looked at me and then at the wall. Hang on, I silently said to myself, before he hit me, he did the same thing. I looked at the wall and when I saw his wall clock and saw what time was it, I realised we have not moved Jack's clock forward to mark the beginning of summer. No wonder he hit me because it was way too early for him to get up. By the time I came to wake him up it was five o'clock on his wall clock. I sincerely apologised to Jack for not moving his wall clock forward and immediately moved it forward and explained to him the reason why, as if he did not know.

I deserved that right hook. Jack was annoyed to be disturbed in his sleep. He felt betrayed and lied to when he noticed that I came at five o'clock instead of the agreed six o'clock. His behaviour did not come out of a blue, it was triggered by my behaviour. He was defending himself from being abused.

Challenging behaviour is not a normal part of dementia but one of the prominent features of dementia. Some may present with challenging behaviour and some may be as sweet as you can get. We sometimes orchestrate challenging behaviour.

SAMMY explains some of our contributing factors:

Staffing: Overstretched staff leads to grossly anxious residents, unfinished and/or cancelled essential tasks, agitated residents, angry residents and unpleased families.

Abandoned by family and friends: Residents feel betrayed and dumped by their loved ones and put in the hands of strangers, feeling trapped.

Misunderstanding: Dissatisfied, disorientated, "I don't belong here".

Misinterpretation: Residents become annoyed by negative signals. Cultural and language differences.

Yoyo: No breakthrough, all plans getting nowhere (moving back to SQUARE ONE).

Chapter Nine

"I will keep grinding."

"I will keep grinding", this has been cited from none other than the best heavyweight boxer of the world, the humblest of them all, A.J. This may sound weird because I mention here a very fit, enthusiastic, well known, active young man. This is no coincidence. Excuse me for my ignorance because I don't exactly know what he means about that but I will tell you what I think it means – readiness, aiming for perfection, doing the right thing, planning, assessing and managing risks, consultation, open- mindedness, knowledgeable, high-quality performance, purpose-driven hard work, precision, accuracy and up-to-date research. We learn from our heroes because they set the bar, they set standards and they are exemplary.

I am not suggesting that you knock them out in the second round but it would be nice if you embrace them with love, high-quality care, consistency, value them and treat them with dignity and respect. Observing and listening and timing your work is the key. Awareness of dementia and most importantly how to deal with people affected by dementia is essential if not a must.

"Get your hands off the pocket and do something for God's sake".

Sitting in the corner near the rear of her bed Nana seemed more in discomfort. Placing her in that corner was a brilliant idea as the view was good but it's getting dark now and Nana is not a quiet lady. Big brother is watching you.

We are here to be their eyes, ears, hands and legs. Service users are aware of their rights to be cared for and this is exactly what they expect from us and nothing less.

"Why are they not like our girls?"

Betty was sitting on her bed, having a cup of tea. She was being attended by an Asian carer. As the carer was assisting her needs, Betty was looking very annoyed, following every step the carer was taking and finally, she asked, "Why are they not like our girls?" What is that all about Betty? I asked. Our girls are quicker and they know exactly what they are doing, she replied. Seemingly, she was not impressed by the kind of service she was getting from the carer. Is it culture or is it inconsistency? This is a cause for concern as person-centred care approach in care and client satisfaction is a priority.

Trust and relationship building in care goes a long way and can mend these niggling cracks. As it has been mentioned in previous chapters team-work is the key. So many times we hear service users trying to draw our attention to their health and safety, kindness, satisfaction and proper care. If the service users can identify the floppy side and make a real noise about the quality of care they deserve, definitely so are the managers.

The life of a dementia sufferers starts by the time their symptoms are noted, diagnosed and takes a noticeable effect on the client. This is by no means an easy task and absolutely way-off to be welcomed by the client and/or families. The client may not notice the change, some may. "I keep forgetting what I was going to do or say", some will comment.

The people in formal care looking after them should be knowledgeable, prepared, forward-thinking, welcoming, supportive, creative, clear-minded, organised and be hands-on. The list is endless. It is rare that a raw talent can bring about these qualities.

Jan Sawdon of Northumbria University, in their 'Connect with us' says: A resource for care home managers developing services for people with dementia shows how he dug deep training home managers about dementia awareness and how to manage their care homes, developing their staff, paying attention to the dementia sufferers, building a knowledgeable, caring, empathetic and creative team.

In his effort to develop the care home managers he stressed these guidelines:

On Staff Selection

- Be clear in your job descriptions and person specifications, and plan your interview to draw out the qualities you need.
- Arrange for a potential member of staff to spend time in the home meeting residents and staff, gauging their response with people with dementia can be part of the process of selection.
- Ask how they would approach a situation using real examples that you have experienced.
- Involve your most aware staff in the interview process.

- Remember that sometimes someone with no experience can demonstrate empathy and warmth, can a real find.

On Staff Retention:

- Be person-centred in the support of your staff.
- Recognise and praise good practice immediately.
- Recognise the complex skills they will be using and the emotional impact they will experience.
- Ensure good systems are in place for supervision where staff can be supported to bring real problems and have them addressed.
- Have a good written sickness and absence policy, perhaps with a reward structure built-in, that you follow consistently.
- Consult with staff at all levels regularly about all aspects of care and the home, and recognise and draw on their ideas and involve them in decision making where possible.
- Ensure your senior staff are providing the same person-centred model of care to residents and staff over the twenty four hour period and monitor this.
- Recognise the special overnight care needs for people with dementia and ensure night staff are provided with the skills and support to meet these.

On Staff Development:

- "Walk the walk" with your staff. Be on the floor for part of each day modelling a person-centred approach.
- Encourage the use of imagination and creativity in your staff.
- Make use of handovers to encourage sharing of knowledge and raise topics for discussion.
- Be opportunistic so that every situation can be a learning experience.
- Organise home-based, ongoing training for staff.
- Use training packs provided by organisations such as the Alzheimer's Society and videos to trigger discussions.
- Access distance learning approaches through local colleges where the learning is focussed on personal experience of working with residents.
- Develop your own training that is tailored to the needs of your residents. There are "training the trainers" courses available.
- Invite in a trainer from the Alzheimer's Society and share the costs with the neighbouring home. This also provides opportunities to learn from each other.
- Following each training, ask each staff member to identify at least one change in practice, however small, and monitor this through observation and supervision. Lots of small changes can have a real effect on the services for your residents.

*

Managers are the captains and are the ones on the driving seats. If they are well equipped and knowledgeable, so should be their staff, and up goes the quality of care.

Much to an urgent need to ensure that those vulnerable residents are safe and secure, managers had to make an informed decision to introduce the use of telecare systems in their homes. Technology plays an important role in improving the quality of life and increasing the safety aspects of care in care homes. Dementia sufferers, due to ageing and other health-related challenges do not only have problems with their memory, but other impairments as well, for example, sight, hearing, sensory movements, moving and handling issues and communication. Their safety is compromised.

The introduction of telecare in care homes has answered some of the concerns which have been bugging the carers for decades. Various measures have been taken, like movement sensors, door sensors, sensor mats etc. have proved to improve the safety of the service users. One of the most intriguing devices which proved vital for communication is the video conferencing device. It not only improved the distant communication but also has been useful in care plan reviews, risk assessment and risk-management. Families who live miles away from the care sector were given opportunities to communicate with their loved ones when this system was put into practice in some institutions. It brought about that connectedness, that feeling of being wanted and loved and teamwork boosted to the service users and trust to the staff looking after them.

Having working systems in place do not only provide safety of the service users but builds up the confidence as well. If the service users know and trust the system, they feel at ease, do not think but know that the staff looking after them will do their best to ensure that they are without a shadow of doubt, safe. Lots of misunderstandings are addressed by availability of resources, good all-round communication, intent, knowledge and ability to all parties including the service users.

Some people do not see it fit for service users to be empowered with enough knowledge about the equipment they are using. The truth of the matter is, these are their equipment and they have every right to know what they are for. Of course they will forget time and time again because of their impairment but you will be surprised as the ins and outs of memory go, how useful the information rendered to them is utilised. Mr Pysio called his sensor mat a spy. Asked why he calls it a spy he said, "every time I make a move to look for something or go to the toilet, there comes a carer, uninvited". On the other end, Renia will rip it off and throw it under the bed because it is disturbing her and does not know why it is put there. The difference of opinions between the two is merely due to the fact that if they do not know anything about it they won't know its use. And that can put them in danger.

They would not know, is not the positive, person-centred care approach as the old saying, "SEE ME, NOT THE DISEASE". There has been a far cry for this change for decades. Change, as simple as it may sound, is not an easy fix. Despite pressures, charities, hospices, volunteering organisations and other social care organisations continue to pioneer some of the innovative approaches to person-centred care.

Chapter Ten

"I cannot talk when I cannot hear."
This sounded very stupid to those who were listening with their ears only but sounded sensible to those who were listening with their hearts and open minds. It made sense, but those in attendance seemed to miss the point. They thought of raising their voices and practising all the skills they have, coming closer, trying non-verbal cues, closing adjacent windows and doors to curb the noise. The lady was becoming more anxious and probably frustrated by this situation she found herself in. "You do not get it, do you", she snapped. "We don't know what you are on about Mrs Vangayo, we will come back to you when you are settled". "Settled? What do they mean by that?" Good thing that she did not hear that one, that might have upset her, I silently thought to myself.

It was around eight o'clock at night, Mrs V. had just finished her usual routine, a quick shower before bed, cleaning her nushers (aka teeth), changing into night attire, television off (time for myself, enough of the world news, she always say when she turns off the television set or the radio), removed the borrowed(hearing aids and glasses) and leave the gifted (wedding ring) and lie down in bed pondering about the day's "cryables, wonderables and laughables" and drift down to the dreamland.(Such is life)

Right at the beginning of this journey, "This is me", a document by the Royal College of Nursing and Alzheimer's Society says, "this document will help you help me in an unfamiliar place". When things are displayed, there is a specific reason for that, it could be educational, it could be something to draw staff's or public's attention, it could be a caution, it could be a supplement, it could be a joke (a day without laughter is like a sad day in a funeral ceremony). The message is simply: do not ignore notices, make use of relevant documents and know who you are dealing with in detail.

Time wasted is costly and unfortunately never returns. They tried every trick in the book to deal with the situation but they missed the vital missing link, "hearing aids". Mrs V. as she puts it mildly herself is lost without her glasses and hearing aids. That does not take a genius to detect, care planning or whichever document one uses to identify the service user's needs and risk assessment.

"Strangers in my world, halleluja," she grinned sarcastically. "Is there anyone who can be of assistance to me?" she asked. Seeing that there is a congress surrounding Mrs V, the boss came along to see what the matter was and when she found out that there was a break in communication and the resident was not having joy, then the million-dollar question popped out. "Is she wearing her hearing aid?" They looked at each other as if saying, "We'll be damned". The search went on. As if there was a £10 000 prize to who found it first, the place was turned upside down. "I found it", said Luvo, with a very relieved expression.

As they gradually try to assemble the hearing aid, Mrs V sighed with relief and said, "That's more like it, thank God at last someone came to his senses. This is what I was looking for, to be complete". "Where were we", she continued. "We came because you called Mrs V", replied one carer. "Oh, thanks, never mind, I am ok, I will call if I need anything".

The door seemed to have narrowed as the carers dashed for the exit bumping at each other as if they were avoiding the CCTV camera, nearly tripping each other on their way out. Anyone can see from their very disappointed facial expressions. Written all over their foreheads were the words—hearing aids and spectacles have an impact on better communication. Lessons learned it's those tiny margins we miss that brings the house down.

It has become a standard rule that every resident admitted to a care home is assessed for mental capacity, have a standard care plan, is risk assessed and risk-managed and above all deprivation of liberty safeguards (DOLS) are put in place, the list is endless.

We need to empower and engage with our residents. Once again the memory problems come into the picture as one of the features with people suffering from dementia.

Doctor Nori Graham and Dr James Warner (2014), citing useful tips from people with dementia, make it very simple.

- Keep a diary.
- Hang a whiteboard with your weekly timetable and reminders of things that you need to do.
- Put labels on doors and drawers to remind you where things are kept.

- Keep a list of telephone numbers with names by the phone.
- Have a newspaper delivered each day, reading this will help to keep your brain active and remind you of the date.
- Put things like keys always in the same place to increase the chance of finding them each time you look for them.
- Tell your family that you do not mind being reminded about things that you need to know.

When dealing with situations like these, carers should read the reactions of the service users very carefully and accurately. Remember, what you hear and see sometimes is not the real testimony of the events. This is not necessarily the reflection of the real attitudes dementia sufferers may actually have.

As mentioned in previous chapters, dementia sufferers are unique. They react differently to the same situation. They might be in one umbrella body, "Dementia", but they are certainly not sharing the same blanket, nor same thoughts or desires.

Body language can deceive you. One of the most serious errors one can make is to interpret a solitary gesture, in isolation of other gestures or circumstances, for example – head shaking and nodding, head shaking means no, and head-nodding means yes. This is not the case in Bulgaria, it is the other way round, head shaking is Yes and nodding is No, that is culture at its best and communication for you. Head scratching on the other hand can mean different things, he/she might have dandruff or fleas, or thinking what to say, or forgot something, or lying. Take a pick, but do not be judgemental. It is a very powerful tool as the spoken languages. It has meaning, sometimes it may be concealed to the observer but knowing your resident is key, that is where effective care planning and good use of multidisciplinary teams come into play. Health care is blessed with the best support system you may ever dream of.

Chapter Eleven

"I am going mad."

She looked very terrified. "Is it raining, it sounds like heavy rain. I must be really going mad", Nong sounded as if she was starting to have incontinence of speech. It was a very calm, warm evening. Most of the people were preparing to retire to their bedrooms except the young at heart who were either out or preparing to go out.

I went into someone else's bedroom. I thought it was mine. I saw this little girl (around 18, I thought) in my bed. I hit her. They told me it was a 93-year-old woman, I am 90 myself, I feel so bad. I believe in Jesus Christ and God is my saviour. She was beginning to be restless and seemed very uncomfortable in her bedroom.

"Can you put me there, please?" She continued and pointed to the wheelchair. "I really need to go out", she said. I rang my colleague for assistance. We assisted her to the wheelchair as she wished. I wheeled her around the corridor, and she asked to stop by the nursing station. "I want to see the doctor, someone please pick up that phone and call the doctor", she demanded. "Let us wait for the nurse in charge and see what her opinion is Nong, shall we", said the carer. Nong was not happy with that but decided to give it a go. As the team was starting to weigh options, she started talking about her past life. Actually, that was very interesting because it was so detailed she could even remember the dates of the events, peoples' names and even quoting other peoples' responses. She sat on her wheelchair for about twenty minutes and she decided to go back to her bedroom.

As soon as she entered her bedroom she started hearing the rain again and this time she mentioned her daughter who passed away two to three years ago and asked why God took her away from her. She started sobbing this time.

Did she have this problem prior to admission? Going back to the famous "This Is Me" and other documents that other homes use for example life history, my life etc, it is very important for carers and professionals to pay attention to the information portrayed by these documents. If clarity is needed, further investigations may be done to relevant institutions or practitioners.

Gathering information and having enough to make a decision and planning treatment is empowering and makes life very easy for both the professionals and the service user and to the joy of the significant ones and the families.

History taking does not only involve the medical history. Lifestyle, previous or recent exposure for example substances at work, incidents at work; be it physical or emotional, domestic issues. That clutter building in someone's brain may have an impact in the later stages of life.

Relevant tests, recent or previously taken may prove to be useful, they might need repeating if professionals, doctors, psychiatrists, microbiologists, therapists deem it necessary to do so.

Remember the first contact is you, the carer/the nurse and without you reporting and/or giving feedback to the nurse (you carer) and the multidisciplinary team (you the nurse) these changes might go unnoticed. What a pity. What an opportunity missed if that happens.

Unfortunately the loser is not the carer, nor the nurse but the one we are looking after, the service user; the one we promised to prioritise and to render safe. Every little detail does matter, that could be the missing link. In science they say small and significant action can have vast far-reaching consequences.

Support for the dementia sufferers should start from the initial stages of diagnosis as these are the scariest times of one's life.

Things To Consider: This Is a Bitter Journey.

Initial stages – Scary, anxious moments, disbelief, difficult to cope.

Confirmed diagnosis – hopelessness, denial, fear of the unknown, shattered

Plan for care – unfamiliar territory, feeling of defeat, loss.

Admission – no man's land, lost, trauma/ family apart, struggling to settle.

Where to get professional help?

Support systems nationally and worldwide are blessed with experienced and capable professionals ready to be of assistance. They are equipped with relevant tools and resources. Here are some individuals, professionals and organisations that might be of assistance.

The pyramid of care and support:
You
NICE
Age UK
Therapists
Local GP's
Dementia UK
Social Workers
Alzheimer's Society
Clinical Psychologists
Dementia Support Groups

Chapter Twelve

"It is too much."

"It is too much", and then she was quiet for a few seconds. "This is too much for me", Marge sounded defeated. "I just want to jump into the lake", she sobbed. "I think I am giving you too much to do instead of sorting myself up", she continued.

As I was listening, something told me to let it flow. I just looked at her attentively, showing a vast interest in avoiding to deflate or disturb her intentions to open up. I had that feeling, should I interrupt her, she would bottle up and not let her feelings go. Remember, a problem shared is a problem halved, so my intentions were to reduce the burden and set her free. No one lives in a shell, the more people communicate, the better the understanding of the situation. Sharing views and getting advice is simply the way to go.

"I do not feel myself, I have lost something, I do not know what, I don't have power anymore", she continued. "How long am I going to depend on other people?" Marge exploded.

What I gathered is that Marge is physically and emotionally on the downward trail and yet she is determined to push herself to the limit. She is a lady who is determined to go that extra mile in everything she does. She knows no limits and to her enough is just a six-letter word produced by an enthusiast and old is "Only Lie Down", get a rest, get up and get on with it. That's determination for you. When the body is worn down only the brave heart tells the story, if it weakens the battle might be more challenging e.g. loss of power, suicidal ideations, loss of confidence, dependence, fear of unknown, anxiety, blaming the other party, challenging behaviour, attention-seeking behaviour or even blaming and asking "why me" questions to God.

Dementia affects people in different manners. Here is how Christine Bryden (2005), portrays the picture:

"As we speak, gaps in the flow of words appear. In our head, a string of pictures has formed, but the words for those pictures no longer make their way into our consciousness, let alone to our mouth. The words for those pictures seem as if they are on a loose spinning wheel. If interrupted, I have to start again, or I simply forget totally what I was going to say. And the thought does not come back later – it is gone for good.

My sentences have become more convoluted as I struggle to find the right word, and if the wheel spins too far, the wrong word comes out."

Our intervention, irrespective of the motion/emotion put in front of us, we need to be clear, sure, professional and confident about our response. As mentioned in the previous page, help is at hand, use available resources and even go beyond if you have to as long it is acceptable and legal.

Inclusion

This is not an easy decision to make. Decisions in care must not be made at face value. A lot has to be considered before a nod is given even if that has to be done under careful supervision. According to Tom Kitwood (2005), "The need for inclusion comes poignantly to the surface in dementia, perhaps in so-called attention-seeking behaviour, in tendencies to cling or hover, or in various forms of protest and disruption. In the ordinary setting of everyday life, it is very rare for people with mental impairments to be included with ease."

The notion of calling dementia sufferers "babies" as they were previously referred to, has taken away their independence and made them more vulnerable, not intentionally at times but people looking after them felt they need be their mother or father figure, doing everything for them rather than including them in their care.

There may be different ways to ensure inclusions but care must be taken because whatever we do must be in line with the person's best interest. As mentioned in the previous chapters, every case is unique. Necessary steps need to be taken to reach the final decision. A team of health care professionals and other appointed significant others qualified to make the decision on the mental capacity of the individual. This is a very crucial procedure and necessary before we put an individual to test. As stated in the basic principles of individual assessment "… the purpose for which it is needed can be as effectively achieved in a way that is best restrictive of the person's rights and freedom of action."

Mental health capacity assessment is done as standard in other care sectors with accepted legal guidelines. The inclusion of staff should not start when problems start to surface but at the initial stages of accepting the residents to care sectors. One of the responsibilities of managers is to lead the performance of the team and the individuals within it by agreeing on objectives and strategies, setting out plans and methods of working, monitoring and evaluating progress and providing a structured approach to care management. By the time they go to assess these residents for potential admission to their homes the stage is set for them to start their assessment considering the client's feelings and emotions, understanding the individual's strengths and abilities, the impact of other people and physical environment, identification of need expressed through behaviour, balancing the requirement of legal risk assessment with a person-centred approach.

On Planning the Care

Managers should consider how to address the person's feelings and needs, provide meaningful activities to enable them to have control over their lives and understand that the behaviour of a person with dementia may express a need rather than a direct result of the disease process, work towards a common philosophy and common goal, assess what the person is able to do, focus on important areas of the person's life. There are some things we tend to overlook in people's lives. Let us pay attention to Renee and Bee and see how superstitions can play a vital role in inclusion and care planning.

Renee: "I grew up very superstitious, thanks to my mum. Love changes things. My mum believed a clock that is not ticking is a dead clock and brings about bad luck. In my life I never had a clock, even a wristwatch without a second hand. The most important thing, it must show life – it must tick. Bee could not stand a ticking watch or a drop of a leaking tap. That drove him potty. I was drawn between giving up any watch in my house or risk losing Bee. We worked it out together. The solution was, we do need clocks, so we cannot get rid of them. Let us get rid of the noise, so we ensured that our clocks were not ticking."

I had to make a choice and quickly. Love won. Bee: As mentioned before, he hated ticking clocks. As time went on he declined to go out of his bedroom even during meal times. He continued with this behaviour declining even essential services like activities programmes. Bee would go willingly with family members and friends to the garden or anywhere except the communal areas. He was referred for help but doctors did not see any signs of being depressed. It was entirely his choice. But the question was, were there clocks on the communal areas? Was there anyone aware of Bee's likes and dislikes?

Reminiscence

As mentioned in chapter one, the history of the resident's life plays an important role in this psychological intervention. As much as it is a very painful adventure for the families, they need to play a big part in this or they have to dig deep into the positive bits of the resident's history or their most recent memorable interests, things that mattered most to them or any useful information that could help jog up their memories a bit. Care must be taken not to upset them or make the situation even worse than it is. This is not A, B, C by any means as memory lapse is unpredictable. This needs careful, structured planning, that is agreed time frame, strategy and agreed role players. Precision is paramount. We need to ride the waves of positivity, sing sweet sounds of hope and show that visible determination of strength to gather momentum. It is time not to follow the trend but to build your own trend.

As mentioned before, the services must be designed around the service user's needs. The healthcare team and families must aim to support and assist the service users to live their lives to the fullest. Empowerment will give an edge to the knowledge and know-how to achieve his/her goals. Not all service users benefit from this procedure, hence a need for a proper assessment. Depending on the severity of dementia, strategic skills may be different. The more severe the disease the slimmer the chances for progress as memory fails more often and retaining the information becomes problematic. Patience and thorough observations are the key elements to focus on.

Chapter Thirteen

"Stop pressurizing me, I know what I'm doing!"

She came to the communal area with such high confidence, I thought she was either a visitor or a relative who came to get her loved one for a special occasion and hey, she was a cutie with a dazzling smile (celebrity style).

She went to the kitchenette and made herself a cup of tea and waited. A carer came along and offered her a bowl of cereal and later a plate with a boiled egg and a slice of brown toast and bacon. She thanked the carer and got on to business.

It was around 07h00 in the morning and most of the service users were still in bed. She finished her breakfast and as she took her cuppa, she reached for her handbag with the other hand and took out her mobile phone, switched it on and dialled. "Hello, did you get my e-mail?" She asked with a broad smile. "Yeah, I sent it last night. I am just finishing my breakfast and after that I am going to assist your dad." "Stop pressurizing me, I know what I'm doing!", she snapped. Sorry about that, she apologised to us, it's just my daughter- I hate to be patronised. There was silence, a deafening silence. She flushed her drink down her throat, cleared the table and went straight through to the bedroom area.

She came with a tall gentleman, hand in hand – almost brushing his left hand with her right hand. She directed him to where she was sitting. Can I have breakfast for my husband, please? She asked politely. She was in control, pure undoubtable control. The carer brought his breakfast, two Weetabix in a blue square bowl, a small white oval jug of milk, sugar in a small silver pot and a small silver crafted teaspoon. The carer assisting was just about to scoop sugar and asked him how many sugars was he taking when…. "He is capable of serving himself, let him do it himself", said the lady. "We are just normal people, you know, we ain't different."

The staff, new and old, permanent /regular, temporary/agency staff must be made aware of the capabilities, likes and dislikes of the residents they are looking after to minimise embarrassment and clash between the two parties. All participants must be familiar with the standard procedures of the home such as mental capacity assessments, the status of the residents (mental capacity) and the need to act at their best interest.

Here are some of the few tips to follow:

Mental Capacity Assessment is divided into two stages.

Stage 1

Ask yourself, does the person have an impairment or a disturbance in the functioning of his mind? For example dementia. This information will be clearly recorded in the medical file/clinical history of the resident by the diagnosing doctor or psychiatrist. If not sure, consultation with the relevant professionals is advised, hence the decision for mental capacity is not a solitary decision. People with mild dementia tend to thrive better than those with profound dementia and live a normal life and can make simple decisions without assistance. Confusion and memory lapses play a vital role in determining mental capacity. Care must be taken to distinguish between the two. The golden rule is not to assume but to make sure necessary steps are taken to reach the correct decision, no rushed decisions.

Stage 2

Go back to your findings in stage 1 and carefully analyse them. Does the assessment determine that the person is unable to make a decision when they are required to make one?

Please note the following:

A person is unable to make a decision if they cannot, understand relevant information about the decision to be made. This is not about ignorance, but understanding simple standard procedures or information processing; retaining that relevant information into their mind; weighing up and using that information as part of the decision-making process and finally communicating their decision by verbal or non-verbal means.

Capacity is not determined by verbal means only. Some people communicate using nonverbal cues. For example, visually impaired people may communicate using braille and hearing impaired may use sign language or written communication.

Suitable resources must be made available to people or referral to relevant institutions made for further investigations. Decisions made by the professionals should ensure that it encompasses their best interest. This will be accomplished by: Giving them equal consideration and non-discrimination

- Considering all relevant circumstances.
- Permitting and encouraging participation.
- Considering their feelings, values, beliefs and respect their views

Home to home as it is often referred to, does not quite look and feel the same. Some service users have that sense of being imprisoned, rendered powerless, their decisions questioned, independence taken away and never being free.

Nan was amazingly the oldest in the care home. She was called Nan because she proved to be everyone's granny wherever she was. She had plenty of time for everybody and everything, shall I say, be it a cat or a dog, a child passing by or her own grand and greatgrandchildren, other residents or staff, I mean everything that walks and talks including teddy-bears (she would talk to them and assume they were walking and talking). She was so adorable, a real lady, looking after everybody's wellbeing. Nan had a remarkable sense of humour. But there was something about Nan – she was never an easy lady. You must really have a very good reason to pass her ideologies. She was smart, reasonable at times and rarely took no for an answer. She was persuasive and sometimes would agree, she has been a little bit naughty and a laugh it off. She liked company, but if she was not comfortable with you she would tell you straight away. She was fearless, she was polite. Dementia has robbed us of this wonderful creature, a blockbuster of a lady. She was one of those residents who was well-loved by all staff and even visitors or shall I say by all walks of life. Sometimes staff would forget that she is over 100 years old (102 to be exact), by staying with her most of the day and sometimes night and being sad when she wanted to go bed -she was such a pleasure to be with.

It was around 22h45 on a very cold night and almost all residents except Nan had already retired to their bedrooms. Nan, as usual, was sitting on her comfortable reclining chair, drinking her cup of tea. She was noticeable staring at the wall filled with pictures, notices, decorations, calendars, handmade work of art from both staff and residents. Nan shook her head and let out a very deep sigh and said, "Oh, I do not blame him". "Nan, what are you talking about?" asked the carer who was looking after her at that time. "Poor man, he is running away from dementia accredited home", replied Nan sounding very concerned. She was still staring at the writing hanging on the wall and the picture below the writing.

There was a square-like portrait on the wall written in blue on a white background: This home is dementia accredited and just below that (separately though), there was a picture of one of the residents in his heydays, playing football. He was really in good shape, controlling the ball with his feet whilst running. Nan put 2+2 together to reflect what she was really thinking about the services.

As mentioned in the previous chapters, the assessment of the mental health capacity goes along with further assessment and compliance with the deprivation of liberty safeguards and all the perks going along with all required procedures and implementation of such.

Chapter Fourteen

"A stranger in my house."

It was a rather busy night. We had just finished the security checks and everyone who needed drinks were served according to their choices. The carers collected the used cups and jugs to do the washing up and refill the jugs with fresh water for the night. A doorbell rang. "At this hour?" asked Mary-Ann, rather astonished. "Be careful, this place is spooky", said Julius giggling. "Answer the bell, I am not going near that door", said Mary-Ann backing away from the door. "Let us not keep the devil waiting in case he becomes angrier and angrier", said Julius jumping off the chair and heading for the door.

As he opened the door, a tree of a man stood still with his big black and white cap, a mobile phone and a body camera on his chest, wearing all black with a dark blue armour vest and black shiny shoes, a typical officer. "Hello officer", saluted Julius. His voice was full of manners and respect for a change.

"Good evening, sorry to disturb you at this time, I understand you are very busy. Do you happen to have Mrs No-cheecky here?" asked the officer. Julius looked puzzled for a second or two and recovered quickly and finally answered, "Of course, come in officer. How can I be of assistance?"

"We received a call from Mrs No-cheeky at around midnight complaining that there are two strange men outside her bedroom whispering and attempting to enter her bedroom. She described them as one of Asian origin, short and stout and the other one tall and looked African and she swore she never saw them before and definitely not the employees of this home she lives in."

"Oh! Mrs N. She is one of our service users. She reacts strongly to strangers. Hold on officer, I will call the nurse, she is the better person to speak to", said Julius. "Take a seat, I will be back soon".

"I don't mind standing", replied the officer on duty. A short brunette with a polish accent rushed to the lounge where the policeman was standing, bowed and shook his hand.

"So sorry Sir to waste your valuable time. I apologise on behalf of the home, management and staff. It is our fault not to introduce the new agency workers who are helping us out tonight to Mrs No-cheeky. I promise this will never happen again. Our facilities are locked day and night and all our residents are safe and in no danger and visitors at this time are only allowed by the manager's or senior staff's permission/approval."

The policeman thanked her for her time and information and having been satisfied that Mrs No-cheeky was not in any danger he vacated the premises and promised that he was going to record the incident and close the case when he reached the police station.

Nurse Natare thanked him for coming and apologised again for wasting his vital time.

The officer went off and the nurse closed the door after him. She came back in and went straight to Mrs No-cheeky, reassured her and finally introduced /informed her about the agency carers who were on duty that night to help the team looking after them.

Shouldn't I be told things like these in good times? demanded No-cheeky, sounding very cheeky indeed (but rightly so). Nurse Natare apologised for the third time that night.

The environment we live in should ensure the resident's sense of privacy, free movement and safety without any underlying fears or obstacles (unknown to the occupier).

There are various legal measures to be carefully taken to make the environment more safe for the service users, those when considered, impact a person's freedom, choices and contacts. Depending on their mental health status, necessity means to safeguard the service users can be facilitated through application for Deprivation of Liberty Safeguards (DOLS).

Chapter Fifteen

"I want my life back."

Jo is definitely not in a good mood today, commented the staff. "Come on guys, give Jo a break, it's late at night and she needs a rest, she might be tired, it has been a very long humid day. She is entitled to be grumpy like anyone else. Don't you get moody at times?" asked the other carer.

I watched the film, Grumpy old men, a long time ago. "Guys, Jo is not grumpy, she is fuming, she is really angry and there is a seriousness in her voice and she has never been like this before", continued Emma.

"Let's go and see her", I suggested to the team. The whole team stood up. "No, no, no", I waved them down. "I do not think she will cope with all you lot, let us go Zan" (I pointed to the newly elected team leader who was looking after the residents in this wing). She was a newbie and looked a bit shaky but she maintained a bit of composure as the team was all junior carers. As we approached Jo's bedroom, we could hear the walls trying to cope with her bursting anger. We looked at each other as we strode like soldiers towards the room.

Suddenly there was tranquillity in the room as we were nearing the door. She took two strides backwards and sat on her comfy chair. She had steely eyes and was trembling with anger, controlling her breaths as if she will spit venom straight into the eyes of her prey looking from left to right as if she is sizing us. "I want my life back", she exploded. This was loud and clear and Jo meant business. "You people stole my life, you took my independence, you took away my happiness. I do not belong here!" She said very slowly and very firmly. "I belong to my family. Do you hear me?" Jo asked looking at both of us.

"Yes, yes Jo, we hear you", we said almost at the same time. That was not re-assuring and that was not easing the situation either.

"When do I go home? I want to go home, I have been here long enough". Her voice was becoming sharper and sharper and there was meaning and urgency to her words and she demanded answers and she wanted answers not later than "NOW", according to her. We did not have those answers at that moment as we were cautious not to escalate the situation, as at that moment she would never entertain a "NO" for an answer.

She started to pace up and down her bedroom, talking to herself. She was by no means pleased with us and did not appreciate our intentions to keep her in the home and care for her as she thought she would do better at her home than in ours.

"Jo, you are here because we are looking after you and making sure that your needs are met and your wishes are fulfilled." "My wish is to go home and spend time with my family, can you fulfil that wish for me", she snapped at Zan. "I am sure I can get support at home, I have a big family, brothers and sisters, children and grandchildren. Do you want me to count them for you?" There was a dead silence in the room.

This war is not over by any means and there was no way we were gonna dodge those bullets at that moment (I quietly told myself). There was so much at stake and so much to deal with.

According to Price J. (2008), "Memory is sometimes so retentive, so serviceable, so obedient; at others, so bewildered and so weak; and others again, so tyrannic, so beyond control!"

No matter how we look at it, memory is a very beautiful, valuable treasure. Memory is a fascinating thing. It is a strong tool. Memory lapse in dementia is quite daunting and challenging, be it a short or a long-term memory deficit. It not only becomes a challenge to the carers and professionals but also becomes a worrying, troubling time for the families and significant others of the dementia patients deprived.

When someone who is suffering from dementia is under the spell of his/her memory, it could be two-fold – either entertaining, or all hell breaks loose. The latter is the worst nightmare for the professionals, carers, and even the family members, not to mention the other vulnerable service users. There are the story-tellers and fortune-tellers. Story-tellers are worth listening to. They suck you in and take away your empathy and put the S in it, leaving you with Sempathy (aka Sympathy – is that right?) They give that wow-factor, you start to doubt the doctor's diagnosis and feeling sorry for the situation they are in., but do not prolong the excitement as it can be sour as the time goes. Fortune-tellers can grill the past and dwell on what could have been. Everything to them at this stage has a nasty taste, keep your physical distance and maintain your emotional mileage. They can be challenging, they demand answers- not later than NOW.

That agility and that determination to sift out the truth (according to the resident) produces more frustrations, partially breaks the confidence amongst participants and rocks and tears that trust apart. It causes mayhem as it throws a feeling of guilt to the family and significant others. It is an unbearable sight.

The upbringing, the history of events surrounding your life plays a big or shall I say a vital role in your later stages of life. It's easier to forgive than to forget. Sometimes the exposure to similar or recallable events brings back flashes. They might be vivid or might be as clear as a 60cm Toshiba television screen pictures. These might be exciting moments, recited with joy, shedding those tears but the crucial part is where they are leading.

That's the scenario to normalize before it gets out of hand. How we do it, remains to be seen, as every step we take is as important as the first step we introduced – "fragile, handle with care".

Let us not forget that these memories are emotionally overwhelming not for the residents per se, but to the family members and the professionals as well. Reactions must be carefully chosen – if there is such a thing as taken with an inch of salt. Be careful not to create two worlds in one continent. Memory shapes lives. It creates opportunities and widens horizons. It is a gem, a very treasurable gem. A gift from God.

Deprivation of Liberty – Cited from Alzheimer's Society

"Sometimes caring for people with dementia involves reducing their independence or restricting their free will in some way. If they are receiving care in a hospital or care home, their routine may be decided for them and they may not be allowed to leave. If the person has not freely chosen where they will live in order to receive care, or the type of care that they receive, it is possible that the care will take away some of their freedom. In some cases, this may amount to 'deprivation of liberty'".

This is not always a bad thing and it is often necessary when caring for someone, but it should only happen if it is in the person's interest.

Who wants to live a life that does not guarantee freedom? Few, no not a chance – none.

Life in institutions may not be as dull as one might think. Measures to make sure that this is not as painful as one might think, are in place. Depending on the severity of the disease, with resources in place, service users are allowed to go out with staff members (under strict supervision) or with their families as long as it is safe to do so and guidelines are followed as per deprivation of liberty safeguards. Care homes are flooded with support from pro-dementia services, various health care organisations, legal departments, volunteering organisations and other related services.

Care homes are fast progressing and up to the challenge. The investment in training the staff in dementia care is actually a must when you have people suffering from dementia in your home. The work done by the Alzheimer's Society, Dementia UK and other associated organisations in offering training and running dementia awareness training has drawn an interest in families who have their loved ones suffering from dementia and even the other interested parties who are keen to learn about the disease, its care and its legalities.

Other Things to Consider:

Each person's needs, feelings, desires, choices and beliefs must be a fundamental consideration in any decision making that is centred amongst their lives.

Conclusion

"I think we will get there, Noma Kanjani (no matter how)."

Sooner or later the suffering is going to be contained if not cured. Studies have shown that there is a host of people and organizations that are dedicated to people and families with dementia. Dr Tom Smith (Living with Alzheimer's Disease) also explores how the disease progresses, existing treatments, how you and your family can plan for difficult times, how to deal with each milestone etc. Ongoing research on dementia indicates that help is not that far off.

Looking at the attempts of the service providers from the initial stages and through the process of admission throughout the stay, there is hope that with consistency and precision the suffering can be minimised.

Quoting a few, Four Seasons Health Care Ethos of Care stresses their commitment to individuality and transfer of ownership. "'Your Home' – We believe that we work in your home, not that you live in our workplace", and it goes on "We understand that you left your own surroundings and most of what is familiar to you. We want you to feel comfortable in the knowledge that this is your new home, whether it be for a shorter respite to stay or on a longer term basis and we will adapt our way of working where possible to accommodate your individual routine. This is quite heart-warming and is a good foundation for care and in planning a workable, individualized, relevant care planning". More enticing, Methodist Home Association makes it more homely – "date of moving in", rather than the date of admission which really sounds like hospitalisation. The list goes on and homes have different strategies in dealing with the improvement of dementia care.

This move by the Four Seasons Health Care (FSHC) Group has been produced in consultation with a number of service users, relatives and staff.

Christine Bryden, as she put it, "dementia was a shameful disease to be feared or denied, not one to be acknowledged and battled with." But… come on, this lady has leapt every hurdle. The bravery she showed was and is still one of the natural breakthroughs in dementia, the determination, the eagerness to pull through, the astonishing strength. She has been the ambassador for dementia and proved that there is life with dementia.

There might be unreported fruitful cases of dementia, who knows. Some families cope with their loved ones suffering from mild dementia, depending on their resources and/or using the available local resources and support.

Once again attempts by care homes to inject passion on the caregivers has been immense.

Four Seasons Health Care has come out with the ROCK AWARD – Recognition of Care and Kindness (the Star). This encourages the staff in all codes to go an extra mile and certainly increases care quality and promotes consistency. The boys and girls especially with relevant training, support and encouragement, equipment / relevant tools to do the job have a better chance of improving dementia care.

The project of champions – dementia, dignity etc by Skills for Care UK and other relevant participants used by Bristol Care Homes and other homes throughout the UK are the key in improving dementia care and lives of people living with dementia.

Alzheimer's Society as their logo suggests are really leading the fight against dementia.

They have produced a wide range of publications designed to support people affected by dementia, their families and caregivers using social media-twitter, Facebook and e-books. Amongst their publications are symptoms, diagnosis and treatment, living with dementia, caring for a person with dementia and magazine – "Resource for health and social care professionals".

They have also embarked on campaigns to improve access to health services in care homes for people affected with dementia.

Alzheimer's Society has made £50m in the UK Dementia Research Institute. This is a research fund into the cause, cure, care and prevention of dementia and to improve treatment for people today and search for a cure for tomorrow.

The Governance

The Care and Quality Commission (CQC) as regulators play a very good role in ensuring compliance and promoting high-quality care and best practices. Amongst other series of regulations, I have chosen Regulation 20 – Duty of Candour, which is the legal duty of hospitals, community and mental health trusts to inform and apologise to patients if there have been mistakes in their care that have led to significant harm. Duty of Candour aims to help patients receive accurate, truthful information from health providers. Hopefully this regulation will be preached around the world and/or any other similar or relevant regulation be adhered to. This is a very powerful tool without which abuse will still be a concealed monster. This regulation also encourages health providers to act in an open and transparent way, clear, honest, and communicate effectively with patients, carers and their families throughout their care and treatment including when things go wrong. Hopefully there will be a lesson learned and improvements made when homes encourage carers and other relevant participants to adhere to this regulation and other relevant regulations and controls – if you like.

THERE IS A VERY BRIGHT, POSITIVE, STEADY BUT SURE, SHINING LIGHT AT THE END OF THE TUNNEL…

References

1. Dr Bailey A. (2015), Alzheimer's and Other Dementias – answers at your fingertipsfourth edition
2. Stokes G. (2008), And Still the Music Plays – Stories of people with dementia
3. **3.**Atkins S. (2015), Dementia for Dummies a Wiley Brand
4. 4.Dr Bryden C. (2005), Dancing with Dementia – My story of living positively with dementia
5. 5.McCarthy B. (2011), Hearing the Person with Dementia – Person-Centred Approach to Communication for Families and Caregivers
6. 6.Dr Goldsmith M. (2002), Hearing the Voice of People with Dementia – Opportunities and Obstacles
7. 7.Smith T. (2000), Living with Alzheimer's Disease- New Edition
8. Salomon R. (2014), Seeing Beyond Dementia – A handbook for carers with English as a second language
9. 9.Whitman L. (2010), Telling Tales about Dementia- experiences of caring
10. 10.Alzheimer's Society- Publications
11. Four Seasons Health Care – Ethos of Care

12. Commision for Social Care Inspection – Standards of Care
13. 13.Royal College of Nursing – This is me
14. Methodist Homes Association – Residents Personal files
15. National Health Services – Duty of Candour
16. Brown M. (1969), The manager's guide to the behavioural sciences
17. Humble J.W. (1968) Management by Objectives
18. Smith E.P. (1969), The manager as an action centred leader
19. Commission for Quality Care – Regulation 20
20. Henderson J. and Atkins D., (2003), Managing Care in Context
21. Dr Graham N., Dr Warner J. (2009) Understanding Alzheimer's Disease & Other Dementias
22. Kitwood T. (2005) Dementia Reconsidered -the person comes first
23. Hughes J.C. (2011) Alzheimer's and other Dementias

Useful resources
Dancing with Dementia
My Story of Living Positively with Dementia
Christine Bryden
ISBN 1-84310-332-X (pbk.)
Hearing the Voice of People with Dementia
Opportunities and Obstacles
Malcolm Goldsmith
Preface by Professor Mary Marshall
ISBN 1 85302 406 6
Older People and Nursing

Issues of living in a care home
Edited by Pauline Ford and Hazel Heath
ISBN 0 7506 2438 8

Promoting Positive Practice in Nursing Older People
Perspectives on quality of life
Edited by Sharon Pickering & Jeanette S. Thompson
ISBN 0-7020-2080-X

Seeing Beyond Dementia
A handbook for carers with English as a second language
Rita Salomon
ISBN: 978 1 846 19 892 2

And Still the Music Plays
Stories of People with Dementia
Graham Stokes
ISBN 978 18747 90884

Alzheimer's and other Dementias
Answers at your fingertips
Alex Bailey
ISBN 978-1-85959-552-7

Living with Alzheimer's Disease
Tom Smith
ISBN:0-85969-956-0

Hearing the Person with Dementia
Person Centred Approach to Communication for Families and caregivers
Bernie McCarthy
ISBN 978 1 84905 186 6